Eyesight And Vision Cure

How To Prevent Eyesight Problems
How To Improve Your Eyesight
Foods, Supplements And Eye
Exercises For Better Vision

By Ace McCloud
Copyright © 2013

I0146441

Disclaimer

The information provided in this book is designed to provide helpful information on the subjects discussed. This book is not meant to be used, nor should it be used, to diagnose or treat any medical condition. For diagnosis or treatment of any medical problem, consult your own physician. The publisher and author are not responsible for any specific health or allergy needs that may require medical supervision and are not liable for any damages or negative consequences from any treatment, action, application or preparation, to any person reading or following the information in this book. Any references included are provided for informational purposes only. Readers should be aware that any websites or links listed in this book may change.

Table of Contents

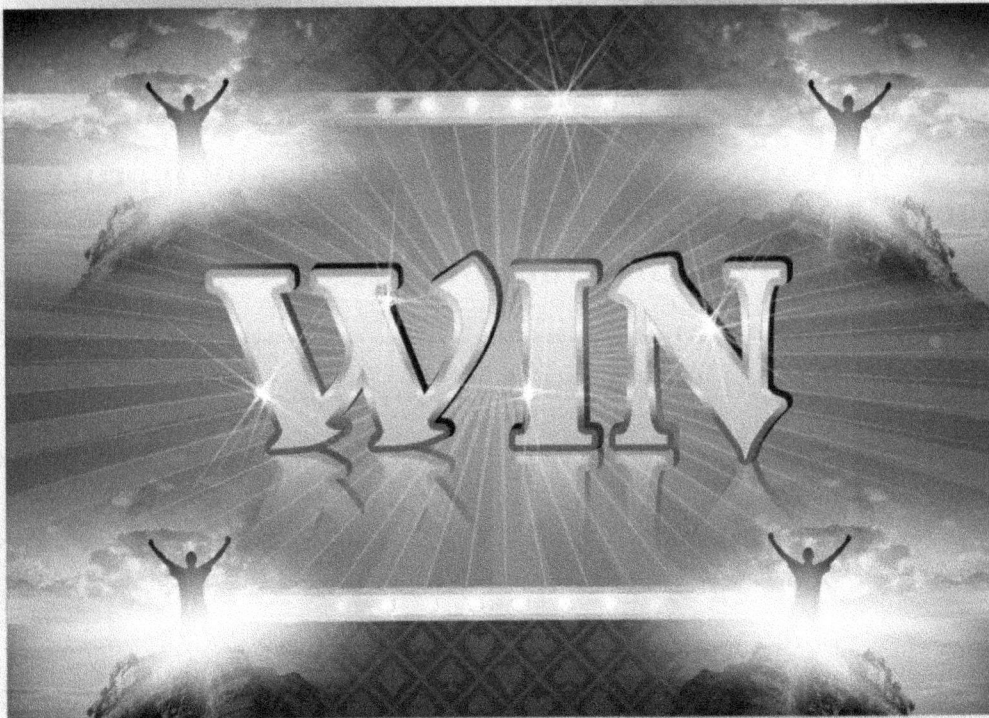

DEDICATED TO THOSE WHO ARE PLAYING THE GAME OF LIFE TO

WIN

KEEP ON PUSHING AND NEVER GIVE UP!

Ace McCloud

Be sure to check out my website for all my Books and Audio books.

www.AcesEbooks.com

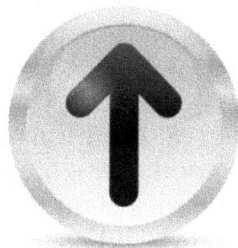

Introduction

I want to thank you and congratulate you for buying the book, *"Eyesight and Vision Cure: How to Prevent Eyesight Problems, How to Improve Your Eyesight, All Natural Foods for Better Vision, And How to Treat Bad Eyesight."*

This book contains proven steps and strategies on how to improve deteriorating eyesight naturally and medically, as well as information on how to prevent your eyesight from going bad in the first place.

If you are concerned about your eyes, the information provided in this book will prove invaluable. If you still have good eyesight, you will learn powerful strategies to keep your eyesight from going bad. If you already have bad eyesight, there is still hope for you. You can still regain good vision. So read on to find out how.

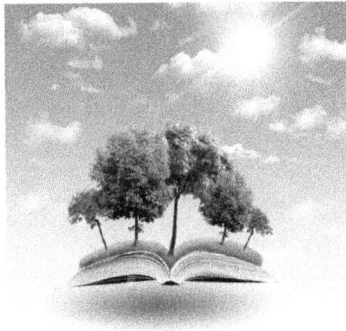

Chapter 1: Causes of Bad Eyesight

The eyes are the windows of the soul. We rely on them in almost everything we do in our everyday lives. Therefore, we need to take good care of our eyes. To do that, we must first know the different causes of bad eyesight.

In our world today, the number of people exposed to things that can cause bad eyesight is increasing, and the longer a person lives, the more they are exposed to potentially eye damaging situations.

Of course, with the advances in medicine, more and more ways have been developed to prevent and cure eye problems. However, this does not mean that a person should neglect their eyesight. On the contrary, we should be more conscious in protecting our eyesight so that it doesn't go bad as we age. Here are some of the most common reasons for eyesight going bad.

GENETICS

Many eye problems are hereditary, passed down through the genes by one or both of the parents.

GLAUCOMA

One of the causes of bad eyesight is glaucoma. It is usually caused by increased pressure within the eye, gradually causing the vision to become impaired.

The two kinds of glaucoma are open-angled and closed-angled glaucoma. Open-angled glaucomas happen slowly and with little pain. On the other hand, closed-angled glaucomas happen rapidly and with acute pain and usually requires immediate medical attention. Both open-angled and closed-angled glaucomas make it harder for the sufferer to see and may eventually lead to blindness.

MYOPIA

Often referred to as nearsightedness, Myopia is one of the most common causes of blurred vision. It is many times genetically handed down, but can also be developed when too much strain is put on the eyes over long periods of time.

HYPEROBIA

Hyperobia, commonly called farsightedness, is typically handed down genetically. It is most often caused by an eye that is too short or a cornea that is too flat, so that images have a tendency to focus on a point behind the retina.

CATARACTS

Cataracts develop in the lens directly behind the pupil of the eye. Overtime, a process called cell turnover occurs, where dubris in the eye builds up over time as cell turnover takes place. This process progresses slowly and clouds the lens, thus impairing vision.

EYE STRAIN

Another issue that can cause bad eyesight is eye strain. In the past, reading was the usual culprit. Nowadays, however, excessive computer usage has replaced reading as the main cause of eye strain.

When your eyesight is used for extended periods of time without allowing it to rest, or if the focus of your eyes does not shift from something near to something far every so often, the eyes become susceptible to losing their ability to focus on distant objects.

This eyesight deterioration usually affects those who spend a lot of time reading, writing, and using the computer.

AGING (PRESBYOPIA)

Aging will inevitably cause one's eyesight to deteriorate. Usually, as people age, their lens becomes thicker and less flexible. The other parts of the eye can also deteriorate over time as well.

Although there are many factors that can cause bad eyesight, there are multiple ways to fight back and keep your vision strong! We will discuss the ways to do this in chapters four and five.

Chapter 2: Contact Lenses versus Glasses

While the goal of this book is to give you ways to improve your eyesight so that you don't need any help from contact lenses or glasses, sometimes you may not have a choice at this period in time. So in this chapter we will briefly discuss the pros and cons to contact lenses versus glasses.

The decision largely depends on you. Some people prefer contact lenses while others prefer glasses, and still others alternate between the two. You need to keep in mind a few things when deciding on whether to wear contact lenses or glasses.

CONTACT LENSE ADVANTAGES

If you are physically active, wearing contact lenses may be a better choice for you during the times that you work out or play sports. Wearing contact lenses during these times will allow you to have total vision and to move whichever way you want without worrying about your glasses falling off your face and getting smashed. In addition, you tend to get better peripheral vision with contact lenses over glasses.

Contact lenses fit directly onto the eyes. On the other hand, glasses have a tendency to slide down your nose because of the oil and sweat from your skin's pores. In addition, you will not need to buy a pair of prescription sunglasses when you are wearing contact lenses.

Contact lenses can also come in different colors so you can change your eye color to match your style or mood. You can dress up your eyes whichever way you want. It can give you a whole new look. There are also contact lenses available with designs on them.

You also don't have to worry about matching your outfit with the color of your glasses, and contacts don't have that annoying reflection that you can get when wearing glasses.

CONTACT LENSES DISADVANTAGES

Since contact lenses sit directly on your eyes, you are at high risk of getting an infection when you do not clean or handle your contact lenses properly. Many people complain about having irritated and dry eyes, especially those who have sensitive eyes. Others have had their contact lenses slip around or off their eyes, causing extreme discomfort.

Cleaning and storing your contact lenses when you are not using them can also be a chore. You need to wash your hands first, take the contact lenses out of your eyes, wash them with your cleaning solution, replace the old solution in your lens case with a new solution, and finally put your contacts into the new solution and in your lens case until you are ready to use them again. This is especially important to do, as there have been cases where people have used tap water to store their contacts, or have failed to wash their hands properly, and have gotten a flesh eating microbe in their eye as a result, causing them to lose vision in one or both eyes.

Putting contacts on can be laborious, especially for people who tend to blink a lot and for people who are new to wearing contacts. Putting some foreign object directly onto your eyes can make you automatically close your eyes while putting them on. In addition, wearing contact lenses can feel uncomfortable since there is "something in your eyes" that wasn't always there.

As you get used to wearing contact lenses and make it a part of your routine, it becomes easier for you to put them on and it will not feel as uncomfortable. However, you will still feel that it is there.

EYEGLASSES ADVANTAGES

For some people, wearing glasses can make them feel or appear to have more character. It can also make someone look more intellectual. There is also a variety of different frames you can buy to complement your outfits and facial structure.

In addition, cleaning and maintaining your glasses is easy. You simply clean them with a soft cloth when dirty and put them on top of your bedside table or in a protective case when you sleep.

EYEGLASSES DISADVANTAGES

Wearing eyeglasses can greatly affect your peripheral vision as the frames of the glasses tend to block your side vision. Wearing glasses may also require you to visit your eye doctor regularly to have your glasses adjusted, as your eyes can get lazy from using the glasses too much and thus your vision can steadily decrease over time. Eyeglass frames also have a tendency to lose their shape when worn on a daily basis, so you may need to consult an eye doctor to have them adjusted.

You will also need to buy prescription sunglasses, which can be pretty expensive, for use in addition to your regular glasses. There are glasses which can turn from clear indoors to dark outdoors, transition lenses, but they are very expensive.

In addition, eyeglasses fog up in cold weather and it usually harder to see with them when it is raining. Eyeglasses can also feel unnatural to wear, since you are adding something to your face that was not originally there.

The choice of whether you will wear contact lenses or glasses is entirely up to you. Do not rely too much on what other people tell you. It is you and not them who will be wearing those things.

Hopefully, however, you will be able to take some of the advice coming up in chapters four and five to eat healthier and do the various eye exercises in an attempt to improve your eyesight or prevent your eyes from going bad in the first place. Another possibility is eye surgery, which can replace your need for glasses or contact lenses all together as well.

Chapter 3: Surgical Eye Treatments

Any surgical procedure that is used to correct problems with your eyesight is called vision correction surgery. It is also known as laser eye surgery. In recent years, great progress has been made in this area. A large number of patients have reported significant improvements in eyesight after having undergone laser eye surgery. Some even say that their vision became even better than before.

Most kinds of vision correction surgery involve changing the shape of the cornea to enable the light coursing through it to be better focused onto the retina. Other kinds of corrective eye surgery involve replacement of the lens.

There are many different kinds of corrective eye surgeries. These include:

LASER IN-SITU KERATOMILEUSIS (LASIK)

This type of surgery is used to improve eyesight in nearsighted and farsighted people and those with astigmatism. The tissue underlying the cornea is reshaped so that it can focus light properly into the eyes.

The difference between LASIK and other eye surgeries is that the surgeon makes a flap in the outer part of the cornea to access the tissue underlying the cornea. A computer imaging procedure, called wavefront technology, may also be used in conjunction with LASIK to create a detailed image of the cornea that helps guide the eye surgeon.

PHOTOREFRACTIVE KERATECTOMY (PRK)

This type of surgery is used to improve the eyesight of mildly to moderately nearsighted and farsighted people and those with astigmatism. A laser beam is used by the eye surgeon to reshape the cornea. The laser projects a beam of pulsing UV light that is directed onto the corneal surface of the eye.

LASER EPITHELIAL KERATOMILEUSIS (LASEK)

This type of surgery is a variant of the PRK. The eye surgeon creates an epithelial flap, and then the epithelial cells are loosened by an alcohol solution. A laser is then used to reshape the cornea. Afterwards, the flap is replaced with a soft contact lens to secure the eye while it heals. This kind of procedure is used to correct the vision of nearsighted and farsighted people and those with astigmatism.

AUTOMATED LAMELLAR KERATOPLASTY (ALK)

This type of surgery is for treating people with extreme nearsightedness and those with minimal degrees of hyperopia (farsightedness). Similar to LASIK, a flap is likewise made in the cornea to allow the surgeon to reach the tissue under the cornea. The difference is that ALK does not require a laser. Rather, one more incision is created on the outer part of the cornea to change its shape.

REFRACTIVE LENS EXCHANGE (RLE)

This type of surgery is also known as clear lens extraction. It is quite similar to cataract surgeries. It involves making a small incision at the edge of the cornea to replace the natural lens with a silicone or plastic lens.

It is also called PRELEX, clear lens exchange, clear lens extraction, and refractive lens replacement. Refractive lens exchange is used in correcting severe farsightedness or nearsightedness.

This type of surgery may be appropriate for those with thin corneas, dry eyes, or other corneal problems. However, other types of procedures are needed to correct problems with astigmatism.

EPILASIK

This type of surgery is similar to PRK. A very thin layer is separated from the cornea and is either left off or replaced. The cornea is then reshaped and the area is protected with a soft contact lens while it is healing.

PRESBYOPIC LENS EXCHANGE (PRELEX)

Presbyopia is a condition wherein the eye's lens is no longer flexible. It then becomes more difficult for the eye to focus on nearby objects. Presbyopic lens exchange (PRELEX) is a type of eye surgery where a multifocal lens is implanted for the correction of presbyopia.

INTRACORNEAL RING SEGMENTS (INTACS)

The intracorneal ring (ICR) segments procedure involves creating a small incision in the cornea and then placing two crescent-shaped plastic rings at the outer edge of the cornea. These two rings reshape the cornea, flattening it to change the way the light rays focus on the retina.

This type of procedure was originally used in treating mild nearsightedness. However, it was replaced by laser-based procedures. Occasionally, irregular astigmatism associated with keratoconus is treated using this procedure. Keratoconus is a condition wherein there is thinning and irregularity in the cornea that could lead to loss of eyesight.

PHAKIC INTRAOCULAR LENS IMPLANTS

Patients who are too nearsighted to have LASIK and PRK procedures can benefit from phakic implants that are inserted through a small incision at the edge of the cornea. It is then attached to the iris and inserted behind the pupil. The difference between phakic implants and RLE is that the eye's natural lens is left in its original place.

ASTIGMATIC KERATOTOMY (AK)

Those people with astigmatism have football-shaped corneas. Astigmatic keratotomy (AK) is a surgical procedure that is used in correcting the vision of people with astigmatism. However, a laser is not used in this procedure. Rather, the surgeon creates a single or dual incision at the area of the cornea where it is most steep. Those two incisions enable the cornea to be more relaxed and become rounder in shape. It is possible to use this procedure by itself or in conjunction with some other types of laser eye surgery.

RADIAL KERATOTOMY (RK)

Radial keratotomy (RK) is a type of procedure that used to be one of the most commonly used procedures in correcting nearsightedness. However, there are an increasing number of successful laser eye surgeries that have been developed, thus making radial keratotomy rarely used these days.

SAFETY AND EFFECTIVENESS OF LASER EYE SURGERIES

The outcomes of laser surgeries involving the eyes have been very promising. However, there are also some side effects that may occur. Therefore, it is necessary for you to know what those side effects are and to keep them in mind if you are deciding whether to undergo laser eye surgery or not. Some of these are listed below:

INFECTION OR DELAY IN HEALING: Less than 1% of people who have undergone photorefractive keratectomy had infections as a result of the procedure. As for LASIK surgery patients, the occurrence of infection resulting from it is much lower. Generally, infection that develops from laser surgeries usually brings about additional discomfort and delays the recovery process.

UNDER-CORRECTION AND OVER-CORRECTION: Accurately predicting the outcome of laser eye surgeries is difficult to do, and you usually won't know the true results until after the eye has healed. Even after undergoing laser eye surgery, it is possible that you may still require corrective lenses. Laser enhancement is done as a secondary eye surgery when the first one results in less than ideal results.

WORSENED VISION: It is rare, but it is possible to have worse vision after a surgery. Some common causes of this include an error in the removal of tissue or excess haze in the cornea.

EXCESSIVE HAZE IN THE CORNEA: Haze in the cornea results from the natural recovery process following laser eye surgery. Usually, it has no effect on the end result following the surgery, but there have been cases where it has turned out to be a problem and negatively affected vision. A follow-up refractive or laser eye surgery procedure may be required to correct this. With LASIK surgery, though, the risk of corneal haze is much lower than that of PRK. In addition, using mitomycin during PRK has proven to be very effective in preventing the occurrence of excessive corneal haze after surgery.

REGRESSION: The effects of refractive or laser eye surgeries can sometimes decrease over some months or years. When this occurs, a follow-up surgery is often recommended to achieve the best results.

HALO EFFECT: The halo effect is characterized by an optical effect that occurs in dim lighting. The pupil enlarges to take in more light. During this enlargement of the pupil, the untreated area outside the cornea gives off a second image.

This halo effect sometimes occurs in LASIK surgery or PRK patients. This can interfere with night vision and night driving, especially among patients with extremely enlarged pupils under dark conditions. The Use of wavefront technology during eye surgery has been found to greatly decrease the occurrence of the halo effect.

FLAP DAMAGE OR LOSS: Flap damage or loss is a rare risk factor exclusively for patients who have undergone LASIK surgery. The hinged flap on the central cornea may require repositioning during the first few days after surgery. On very rare occasions, problems with the flap may occur when the eye suffers an extreme direct injury.

Refractive or laser eye surgeries need healthy eyes that do not have retinal problems, corneal scars, or any other eye disease. Aside from the side effects stated above, some other questions you may want to ask before choosing whether or not to undergo laser or refractive surgery are: Will my insurance cover my laser eye surgery costs? How long will the healing take? Will some of my activities be restricted after the surgery?

Advancements in medical technology have been getting better every year. Therefore, it is very important that you explore all options and possibilities before deciding which eyesight repair treatment is best for you.

LASIK SURGERY ADVANTAGES

The many benefits of LASIK surgery are the following:

- It is very good at correcting your vision.

- It is an almost painless procedure.

- Eyesight is corrected almost immediately or within the day following the procedure.

- It is a non-invasive procedure, requiring no bandages or stitches afterwards.

- A second surgery, called laser enhancement, can be done to adjust your eyesight if needed. You can correct your vision later on with few complications if necessary.

- Most patients no longer require eyeglasses or contact lenses after undergoing LASIK surgery.

LASIK DISADVANTAGES

Although there are numerous advantages in undergoing LASIK surgery, there are also some disadvantages that you need to consider before deciding. These include the following:

- Changes to the cornea that are made during the LASIK procedure cannot be reversed.

- LASIK surgery is a very complex technical procedure. The surgeon may experience problems while cutting the flap and this can have a permanent effect on your eyesight.

- Although this rarely happens, LASIK surgery can cause a patient to lose optimal vision, which is the highest degree of vision one can achieve while wearing contact lenses or eyeglasses.

POTENTIAL LASIK SURGERY SIDE EFFECTS

Some people who have undergone LASIK surgery may experience discomfort during the first 24 to 48 hours after the procedure. Glare and seeing halos around images can also occur. This can lead to difficulty in seeing in the dark, more so when driving at night. Eyesight can also fluctuate. In addition, you can develop dry eyes after the LASIK surgery.

LASIK SURGERY PREPARATION

Before undergoing LASIK surgery, there will be a coordinator who will meet with you to discuss what you can expect during and after the surgery. During this discussion, the coordinator will evaluate your medical history and fully examine your eyes. Initial tests that are done typically include a corneal thickness measurement, refraction, corneal mapping, and pupil dilation.

After this initial evaluation, you will typically then meet with your surgeon. This is a good time to ask them any questions or raise any concerns you may have. After that, and if advised by your surgeon, then an appointment for your procedure is scheduled. Plan to have someone with you to help you get home after your surgery.

If you wear rigid gas-permeable contact lenses, you should refrain from wearing them for at least three weeks prior to your evaluation. Other kinds of contact lenses should also not be worn for at least three days prior to your evaluation. However, if you wear eyeglasses, you should bring your eyeglasses to the surgeon so he can review your prescription.

On the day of your surgery, you should eat a light meal before going to your surgeon. Be sure to take all your surgeon's prescribed medications. Avoid wearing makeup or any bulky accessories that might interfere with your head's position under the laser. If on the day of your surgery you are feeling sick, call your surgeon immediately to determine whether your surgery needs to be postponed or not.

LASIK SURGERY PROCEDURE

A local anesthesia in the form of eye drops is generally used before the surgery begins. Usually, this takes about 10 minutes to take effect. You can also request a mild sedative.

During your surgery, a microkeratome or femtosecond laser is used to cut a thin flap in your cornea. Then, the corneal flap will be peeled back so that the underlying tissues can be reshaped using another laser. After reshaping the cornea to help it properly focus light, the corneal flap is put back to its original position, completing the procedure.

POST LASIK SURGERY EXPECTATIONS

You can expect your eyes to be dry, even though they may not feel that way. Your surgeon will generally give you prescription eye drops to prevent infection and inflammation after the surgery. The eye drops also help your eyes to remain moist. However, these eye drops may also cause a slight burning sensation or blurred vision after using them. Remember not to use any kind of eye drop that is not approved by your ophthalmologist.

Healing usually occurs very rapidly after your LASIK surgery. Your eyesight may be blurred or hazy on your first day after your surgery, but most patients start noticing improved vision within just a few days after the surgery.

Follow-ups after the surgery will vary depending on your chosen surgeon. You will most likely need to revisit your eye surgeon for an evaluation one to two days after your LASIK surgery. You may also need to visit your surgeon at regular intervals during the first six months following your surgery.

Chapter 4: Eye Exercises and other Strategies to Improve Eyesight or Prevent it from going bad

One of the most important of the five senses of the human body is our sense of sight, and about eighty percent of the information we receive is through our vision. For most people, nothing is more important than preserving their sense of sight. Luckily, there are many ways to do this.

In the United States, it is reported that almost 90 million people have problems with their eyesight, and more than 50,000 have lost their vision completely. Fortunately, most eye problems nowadays are treatable. Even serious eye problems that could cause blindness are preventable, especially if the problem is identified and addressed at an early stage.

Restoring poor eyesight naturally is possible if you know what to do. Our eyesight is one of the most precious treasures that we have. Therefore, we need to take good care of it.

It is important to try and improve or restore bad eyesight as soon as you are diagnosed with an eye problem. Here are some of the many ways in which you can naturally improve your eyesight. It is very important to do these exercises on a regular basis. Just like a bodybuilder has to work out many times to gain great strength and muscle mass, you will have to exercise your eyes diligently to get your desired results!

EYE EXERCISES

Taking just 10 minutes of your time to do eye exercises several times per day can be greatly beneficial for your overall vision health. Your eyes should keep changing focus to ensure that the muscles controlling your eyes are exercised and strengthened.

While not all vision problems can be restored naturally, a vast majority of them can be, such as being short or far sighted. While contact lenses and glasses are very helpful, they can make your eyes lazy, thus leading you to get more powerful prescriptions year after year to compensate. Here are some simple exercises you can do almost anywhere.

Palming: Once or more daily, sit comfortably; rub your hands together to make them warm, and then cover your eyes with them for three minutes. Try to ensure that no light gets in and try and visualize something interesting during this time, such as some of the things you would like to be doing with perfect eyesight.

Eye Massage: Sit or lie down in a relaxed position and very gently massage your eyes for several minutes. This helps reduce eye strain and increase circulation. Be sure to be very gentle when doing this.

Presbyopia Exercise: To perform this technique, cross your eyes by focusing on the tip of your nose. Then shift your focus to an object in the distance for several seconds. Do this ten times in a row, take a brief break, then do this again ten more times. Be sure to inhale deeply when focusing on your nose and to exhale deeply when focusing on the object in the distance. This exercise is good for decreasing your chances of getting macular degeneration as well as increasing circulation in the eyes and improving the eyes focusing power. Ideally, this exercise should be done 3-5 times per week.

Moving Target Eye Exercise: Take a pen and extend it out in front of you to arm's length. Focus your eyes on the pen and then move the pen slowly towards your nose, watching it the whole time. Once the pen becomes blurry or you start to lose focus, then close your eyes briefly, bring the pen back out to arm's length, and then open your eyes and change your focus to a distant object. Then repeat the exercise again. Do this technique for several minutes up to twice a day. This exercise strengthens the muscles in your eyes to improve their ability to focus on objects that move from far away to close up.

Eye Strengthening and Improved Focusing Exercises

- Sitting in a relaxed position, roll your eyes in a complete circle, from up, to right, to down, to left. Then repeat in the opposite direction. Continue alternating directions until your eyes feel tired.

- While sitting in a relaxed position, imagine that you are looking at a large imaginary square. Look up at the top right corner of the square, then look down to the bottom left corner of the square, then look to the upper left corner of the square, then down to the bottom right corner of the square. Once this is done, repeat the exercise if the opposite direction. So you'd go from the lower right corner to the upper left corner to the bottom left corner to the top right corner of the square. Do this exercise 10 -1 5 times.

- Close your eyes and squeeze them tightly together. Then open your eyes. Do this exercise 10 - 15 times.

- Focus your eyes on a spot between your eyebrows for 3 to 5 seconds. Then close your eyes and relax for several seconds. Do this exercise 10 - 15 times.

- Sit in a relaxed position facing straight ahead. Without moving your head, look up as far as possible. Then look in a circle, starting by looking to the right as far as possible, then circle your eyes down, and then to the left as far as possible. Close your eyes and relax for around 5 seconds, and then repeat this exercise in the opposite direction, looking up first and then circling to the left, down, and then to the right. Repeat this entire exercise in both directions 10-15 times.

- Sit in a relaxed position and when ready, cross your eyes and stare at the tip of your nose. Keep your eyes focused in this position as long as you can and then close your eyes and relax them for ten to fifteen seconds. When first starting out, just do this exercise 2 to 3 times, and over time, work up to ten or more repetitions.

- Sit in a relaxed position with your back and neck straight, and then have your eyes follow the pattern of a figure eight. Do it in one direction, then in the opposite direction, for several minutes.

- Sit straight while keeping your neck stiff. Have your eyes follow the swinging motion of a pendulum. An easy way to do this is to use your mouse cursor, and follow it in a swinging motion across your computer screen, or attach a small ball to a string, and swing it in front of you, with your eyes following the ball. Do this for several minutes.

- This exercise involves focusing on various objects that are at different distances from you. Trace the outline of these objects with your eyes. Do this exercise for several minutes.

- Start this exercise off by going outside. Look at something in the far distance, at least 1 mile away. Hold this position for 5 seconds. Then look at something around 25 feet away, and focus on it as clearly as possible. Hold this position for another 5 seconds. Then look at something around 600 feet away, and focus on it for 5 seconds. Then lastly, try and find an object as far away as possible and focus on it for 5 seconds. Try and do this exercise several times per day.

- Another good exercise that is good for focusing involves selecting two focal points, one that is very near to you and one that is about 20 feet away. Start by looking at the point that is closest to you for a few seconds, and then switch to the point that is about 20 feet away. Keep switching between the two points while breathing deeply for 2 to 3 minutes.

YOGA EYE EXERCISE

This is a great exercise that you can do to strengthen your eyes. To see exactly how to do it and be guided in your exercise, click on this link that will bring you to the YouTube video, Yoga Eye Exercise on You Tube, by YogaVidya English.

CHINESE EYE EXERCISES TO RELIEVE EYE STRAIN

Start by doing a quick warm up. Move your eyes to the right, then to the left, then up, then down, clockwise, counterclockwise, diagonally from lower left to upper right, then diagonally from lower right to upper left. Do each movement ten times. When done, gently rub the eyes for several seconds.

Next, place the tip of your index fingers or your middle fingers against your temples. Make sure your fingers are even with your eyebrows, and then massage in small circular motions for one to two minutes. Switch back and forth from between small circular clockwise motions, and small circular counterclockwise motions.

Now gently massage around the upper and lower parts of your eye socket in a circular motion using the tips your fingers for 15 to 30 seconds. Then use your first two fingers and thumb to massage the bridge your nose (upper part of nose) for 15 to 30 seconds. Repeat both parts of this exercise from between four to eight times.

Next, close your eyes and press your thumbs to the spot where your eyeball meets the upper part of your eye socket. Use your index or middle finger to pull down on your forehead near the hairline. Do this six to ten times.

The next part of this exercise is to take your thumbs, put them behind your ears, and rub up and down gently for around 30 seconds. Then move your thumbs to the back of your head where the skull meets the neck and rub on either side of the neck for another 30 seconds. Finally, move your thumbs to the back of your head directly opposite of your eyes, and massage and in a circular motion for 30 to 60 seconds.

Do this complete exercise several times per day for optimum benefit. When this exercises is complete, stare at a spot in the far distance to allow your eyes to relax.

For added benefit, you can roll your feet on a rolling pin, focusing on the point between the second and third toes. This is believed to be a reflex point for the eyes.

Another reflex point that is rumored to help the eyes is located in your hands. Take your right thumb and press it into the palm of your left hand about one to two inches in from between your left thumb and left index finger. Then take your right index finger and put it underneath your thumb on the opposite side of your hand and squeeze your finger and thumb together until it is slightly painful. Repeat this process on your other hand. Do this several times then relax.

REST

When working or reading, especially in front of the computer, take breaks every 20 minutes or so to rest your tired eyes. Be sure to focus on something at least 20 feet away for 20 seconds or longer at the beginning of your break. Brief rests between working can help prevent bad eyesight caused by eye fatigue and eye strain. Close your eyes and just relax, rubbing your eyes gently. It has also been found helpful to take a brief walk or to focus on any plants, trees, or natural vegetation in the area. This would also be a great time to do a few of the eye exercises mentioned earlier, or just simply clear your mind and take it easy for several minutes.

BLINKING

Blinking often helps the eyes' retain moisture. Dry eyes can lead to corneal abrasions that decrease the eyes' ability to see. Strong wind or even the air conditioner can cause the eyes to get dry. Cold air is also more effective at drying your eyes as compared to room temperature or warmer air. Try and remember to blink often.

PROPER MONITOR PLACEMENT

The proper viewing distance between you and your computer screen is about twenty-four inches. Try and position your monitor so that it sits directly in front of you, and so that you are looking slightly down at it. Studies have shown that looking up at a computer screen is particularly fatiguing, while looking down at a computer screen is far less so.

Eye strain can result from using the computer for extended periods of time without resting in between. Hence, you should remember the 20-20-20 rule. Every 20 minutes, you should look away from your screen and focus on something that is about 20 feet away from you for about 20 seconds before resuming your work on the computer.

PROPER TV PLACEMENT

Try and keep your TV away from reflective surfaces, such as windows and mirrors that can bounce light onto the TV screen and cause glare. Also, you want your TV at eye level, so that when you are sitting down you don't have to tilt your neck to watch the TV. Do not sit too close to the television. Although it was once rumored that sitting too close to a TV set would cause bad eyesight, the reality is that it will just give you a headache if you are sitting too close. If headaches occur, move further away from the TV screen. A good reference to go by is if your TV is 26-32inches wide, then you want to sit from three to seven feet away. If your screen is from 37-42 inches wide, then you want to sit about five to ten feet away. For screens 47 inches and larger, a good rule of thumb is from seven to fifteen feet away.

SUPPLEMENTS

Supplements are a great way to ensure that your eyes are getting all the nutrients they need. Daily supplements of antioxidant vitamins, flax seed, lutein, and zinc are very helpful in avoiding age-related macular degeneration and cataracts. Also, be sure to include the following vitamins in your supplementation: Vitamin A, Vitamin C, Vitamin D, and Vitamin E. Also, there are supplements that are specifically blended and designed to help with your eyesight. My favorite is OcuGuard Plus from Twinlab, and I would highly recommend taking this or a similar supplement that is specifically formulated for vision. As always, be sure to consult a doctor before taking any new supplementation.

SUN GLASSES

When you are out in the sun for long periods of time, you should wear sun glasses that block out ultraviolet radiation. Sunglasses with a darker hue tend to protect your eyes better.

Also, when out in the sun, wearing a hat with a brim that can properly shade your eyes will be your best defense against the suns harsh rays.

STOP SMOKING AND DRINKING

If you smoke regularly, now is the time to stop smoking if you are even the least bit concerned about your eyesight. Smoking increases the risk of vascular diseases and makes the blood vessels in the body and eyes constricted. If you would like some serious help with quitting smoking, be sure to check out my book: Quit Smoking Now Quickly And Easily.

In addition, excessive consumption of alcohol can be detrimental to the health of your eyes (although it is true that some amount of alcohol can actually help improve your eyesight). Drinking one glass of red wine a day can actually prevent macular degeneration because it is high in antioxidants.

However, most things in excess are bad. People who consume drinks with alcohol on a regular basis are literally starving themselves of nutrients needed for good vision. Heavy drinking can put you in a state of extreme intoxication, possibly causing short-term eye damage, including night blindness and double vision.

EXERCISE

One of the most important things you can do for overall health and well-being is to exercise daily. Even if it is just twenty minutes of walking a day, it will greatly increase your overall health, which in turn will help you prevent all sorts of ailments, including age-related macular degeneration.

EYE EXAMS

It is important to have your eyes checked out if you notice any decrease in vision or other vision problems. One of the best organizations for doing this is the National Eye Institute. This organization does not pay for your eye care, but they can direct you to different programs that are funded by the government or the private sector.

Chapter 5: Foods That Help Improve Eyesight

One of the natural ways that we can improve our eyesight is through a proper diet. Eating the right kinds of food can provide our eyes with much-needed nutrients that ensure better eyesight.

PROPER NUTRITION AND DIET

Eat lots of fruits that are rich in antioxidants such as blueberries and strawberries. Studies show that people who eat greater quantities of fruits have a lower risk of developing age-related macular degeneration (ARMD) than those who eat smaller quantities of fruits. ARMD is the leading cause of blindness in older people.

Eating at least five servings of fruits and vegetables every day, especially those high in Vitamin A and Vitamin E, can help prevent your eyesight from going bad.

Stay away from fried food. French fries and other greasy foods are loaded with free radicals which reduce your ability to retain antioxidants. These antioxidants are our partners in fighting against vision loss. You should also stay away from low quality carbohydrates like sugary foods. There has been new research that suggests that these types of carbohydrates cause a quick surge in blood sugar levels, which may damage the retina and tiny capillaries in the eye over a long period of time.

BILBERRIES

Bilberries have high levels of antioxidants that can help sharpen your vision. They also contain anthocyanosides that can help reduce deterioration of the eyes.

RED ONIONS

Red onions can help prevent bad eyesight because they contain quercetin, an antioxidant that can prevent cataracts from developing.

CARROTS

Our moms always pester us to eat our carrots, and for good reason. Carrots have beta-carotene that changes into Vitamin A after it enters the body. Vitamin A not only helps preserve eye health, but it also helps to build a strong immune system and it promotes healthier-looking skin.

Raw mature carrots are the top sources of beta-carotene. Baby carrots, sweet potatoes, pumpkins, spinach, and other greens also contain healthy doses of beta-carotene.

A few servings of these vegetables daily will yield great results. Carrots are best eaten raw since some of the vitamins and minerals get lost while they are being cooked. You can also toss carrots, spinach, and other greens together and make a refreshing salad or there are a variety of other creative ways to add them into your diet.

TRIO OF B's

Bell peppers (Red, yellow, orange, red, green, Purple), brussel sprouts, and broccoli are excellent vegetables. They contain tons of Vitamin C which is good for both the vision and the immune system. Vitamin C is a powerful antioxidant that fights off free radicals. It is also known for preventing or slowing down the development of age related macular degeneration, cataracts, and glaucoma.

The daily recommended consumption of bell pepper is half a cup, while it is one cup each for brussel sprouts and broccoli. You can mix them up into a salad or stir fry them in olive oil and garlic.

TURKEY

Turkey is rich in proteins and zinc, and tastes great whether it is roasted or in deli-style slices. The zinc in turkey, when combined with other foods high in antioxidants, can greatly reduce your risk of developing ARMD by about twenty-five percent. In addition, it can also help in protecting the remaining vision of people who have been diagnosed with age related macular degeneration.

You must remember, though, that it is harmful to consume too much zinc. Three ounces of turkey provides the right amount of zinc that you need. You can make a mouth-watering turkey sandwich that is healthy, filling, and delicious. You can also put it in salads or make it as your main dish.

SPINACH

Who doesn't know Popeye the sailor? We all know spinach is his main source of strength, but this leafy green is also known for something else. It is loaded with beta-carotene, Vitamin C, antioxidants, and lutein, all of which are good for the eyes. The lutein in the spinach is a nutrient that can help prevent macular degeneration and cataracts. You can combine spinach with olive oil or vegetable oil for faster absorption by the body. Lutein also keeps the eyes safe from oxidative stress. It acts like a sunscreen by absorbing the blue-light intensity. Kale is also a good source of lutein.

FISH

Omega-3 fatty acids will not only help lower your cholesterol, but it also helps protect your eyes against macular degeneration and dry eye syndrome by producing protective pigments for the eyes. Fish like salmon, tuna, and sardines are the best sources of omega-3. One to two servings of tuna per week can easily meet your weekly requirement. If you have allergies to fish or you do not like eating it, you can opt for fish oil or omega-3 fatty acid supplements. Fish that are rich in omega-3 fatty acids can help protect your blood vessels as well as help prevent clots in the eyes. A great Omega-3 supplement is: Kirkland Omega 3 Natural Fish Oil.

OTHER GREAT FOOD ITEMS THAT ARE GOOD FOR THE EYES

Sweet Potatoes, Spinach, Soy, Garlic, Apricots, Kiwis, Wolfberries, Oranges, Garlic, Apricots, Eggs, Dark chocolate, Onions, Pink and red grapefruit, Kale, Green tea, Quinoa, Sunflower seeds, Avocadoes, Peaches, Mangos, Tangerines, Collard Greens, Cantaloupe, Water melon, Honey Dew Melons, and Tomatoes

JUICING

Juicing is an incredible way to get the nutrients you need in a tasty and easily digestible drink. Simply choose your favorite fruits and vegetables from the choices mentioned earlier, then run them through your juicer. The Breville Juice Fountain is an excellent juicer. The combinations of healthy drinks that you can make that are great for your eyesight are only limited by your imagination. I've included a few of the best recipes below, but don't be afraid to mix and match the fruits and vegetables that are your favorites and perfect your own special recipe. Be sure to drink your fresh juice immediately! It loses nutrients over time, and the best time to drink it is just after juicing. I also like to juice after a meal or a few hours after a solid meal. If your stomach is empty, some juice recipes can cause stomach pain as it is being digested.

My favorite

For this recipe, I don't have specific measurements; I just use a good amount of each of the items listed below. You want to aim for about two large glass fulls of juice. I like to combine everything into a large pitcher, then drink it over the next 30 minutes. But smaller amounts of juicing can also be highly effective and save money over the long term.

Spinach, Carrots, Oranges, Green Peppers, Peaches, Watermelon, Cantaloupe, and Tomatoes

This a great drink for eyesight and tastes great!

Here are three more tasty juice drinks that are good for your eyesight:

First Recipe: 2 apples, 1 beet root, 8 carrots, 1 lemon, and 2 oranges

Second Recipe: 6 leaves of Basil, 12 carrots, 1 lemon, and 6 peaches

Third Recipe: 3 large slices of cantaloupe, 6 carrots, 3 oranges, and 1 green pepper

SMOOTHIES

Making smoothies has recently become my favorite way to make drinks. I like not having to throw away so much of the fruits and vegetables, as you do with juicing, and it is significantly less expensive than juicing. However, when I am seriously looking for a boost, juicing will win out every day over a smoothie. The fiber retention in smoothies is a great asset for it, as is the increased variety of foods you can use in a smoothie. For peak performance, I would suggest including both juicing and smoothies in your diet. I am currently using a NutriBullet Blender to make my smoothies, and I am quite pleased with it. It is typical to include water in a smoothie at a ratio of about 40-50%.

My Favorite: Spinach, Green Peppers, Oranges, Tomatoes, Watermelon, and Carrots

First Recipe: 2 peaches, large slice of watermelon, 2 oranges, and 2 carrots

Second Recipe: 2 cups kale, 3 kiwis, 2 peaches, and 1 cup of bilberries

Third Recipe: 2 green peppers, 1 tomato, 2 carrots, 3 tangerines, and 2 mangos

Conclusion

I hope this book was able to help you to know what to do to prevent your eyesight from going bad, and if it already has, how to improve your eyesight and get it back to normal.

The next step is to remember what you have read in this book and apply what you have learned. By reading this far, it means that you are still able to see. **So protect your precious sense of sight!** Whether your eyes are still in good shape or not, it is never too late to take good care of them and show them some love! With a determined and strategic effort, you should be able to greatly increase your chances of living happily with excellent eyesight! Improving your eyesight takes time, so keep at it and never give up!

Finally, if you discovered at least one thing that has helped you or that you think would be beneficial to someone else, be sure to take a few seconds to easily post a quick positive review. As an author, your positive feedback is desperately needed. Your highly valuable five star reviews are like a river of golden joy flowing through a sunny forest of mighty trees and beautiful flowers! *To do your good deed in making the world a better place by helping others with your valuable insight, just leave a nice review.*

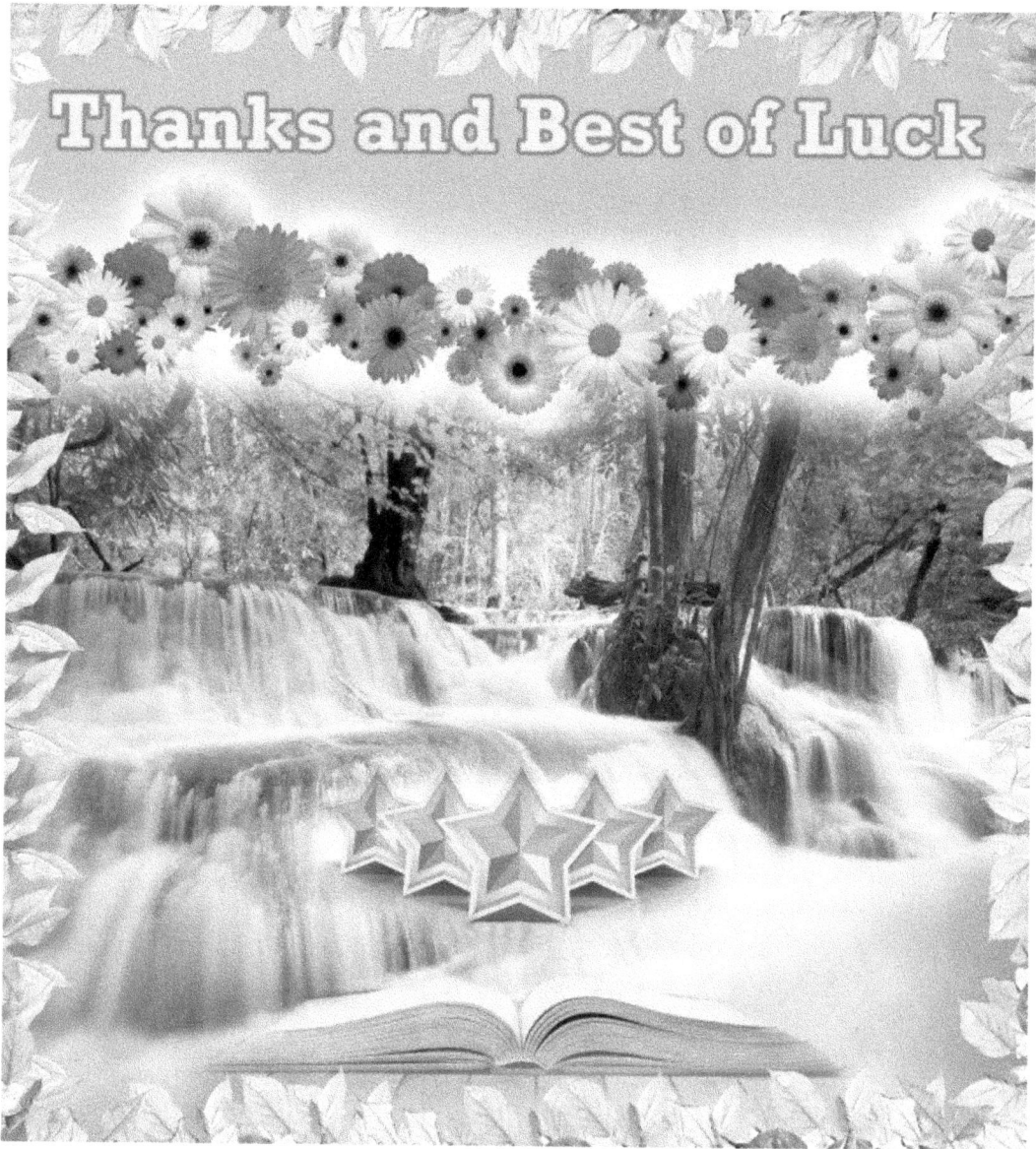

My Other Books and Audio Books
www.AcesEbooks.com

Health Books

ULTIMATE HEALTH SECRETS

HEALTH

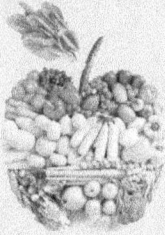

Strategies For Dieting, Eating Healthy, Exercising,
Losing Weight, The Mediterranean Diet,
Strength Training, And All About Vitamins,
Minerals, And Supplements

Ace McCloud

ENERGY
ULTIMATE ENERGY

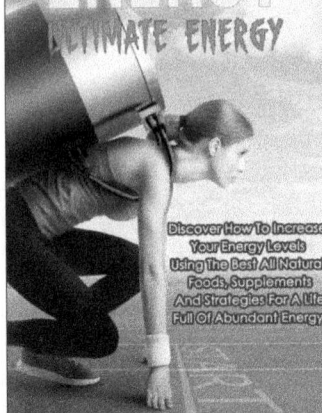

Discover How To Increase
Your Energy Levels
Using The Best All Natural
Foods, Supplements
And Strategies For A Life
Full Of Abundant Energy

Ace McCloud

RECIPE BOOK

The Best Food Recipes
That Are Delicious, Healthy,
Great For Energy And Easy To Make

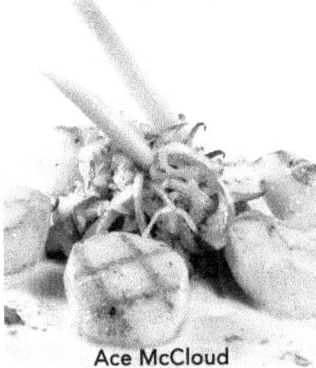

Ace McCloud

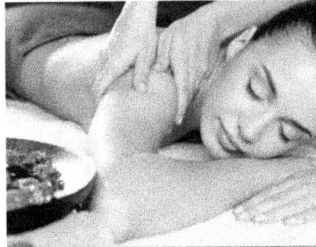

MASSAGE
THERAPY

TRIGGER POINT THERAPY
ACUPRESSURE THERAPY
Learn The Best Techniques For
Optimum Pain Relief And Relaxation

Ace McCloud

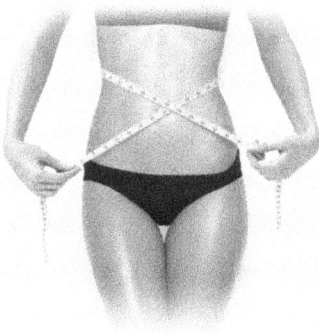

LOSE WEIGHT

THE TOP 100 BEST WAYS
TO LOSE WEIGHT QUICKLY AND HEALTHILY

Ace McCloud

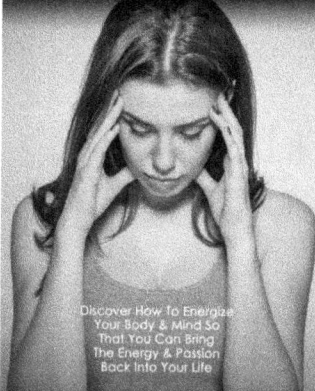

FATIGUE
OVERCOME CHRONIC FATIGUE

Discover How To Energize
Your Body & Mind So
That You Can Bring
The Energy & Passion
Back Into Your Life

Ace McCloud

Peak Performance Books

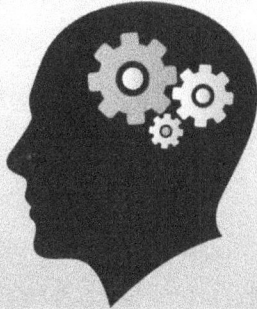

SUCCESS
SUCCESS STRATEGIES

THE TOP 100 BEST WAYS TO BE SUCCESSFUL

Ace McCloud

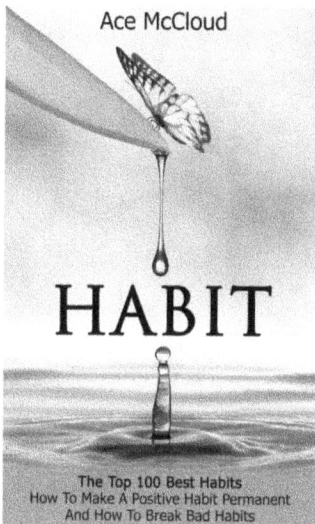

Ace McCloud

HABIT

The Top 100 Best Habits
How To Make A Positive Habit Permanent
And How To Break Bad Habits

MOTIVATION

MASTER THE POWER OF MOTIVATION TO PROPEL YOURSELF TO SUCCESS

Ace McCloud

ATTITUDE

Discover The True Power Of A Positive Attitude

Ace McCloud

SELF DISCIPLINE

Unleash The Power Of Self Discipline, Influence And Willpower In Your Life To Achieve Anything

Ace McCloud

Competitive Strategies

WINNING STRATEGIES

The Top 100 Best Strategies For Peak Performance During Competitions

Ace McCloud

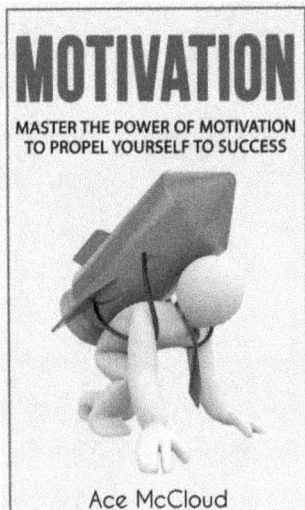

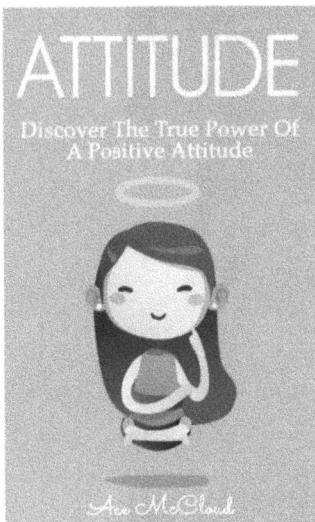

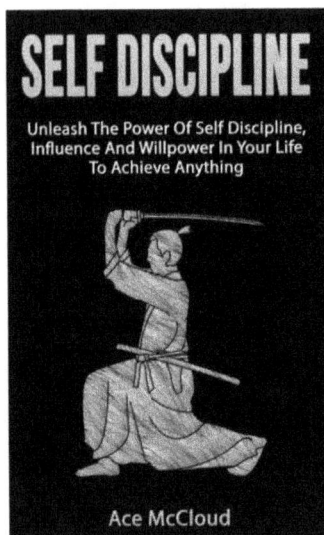

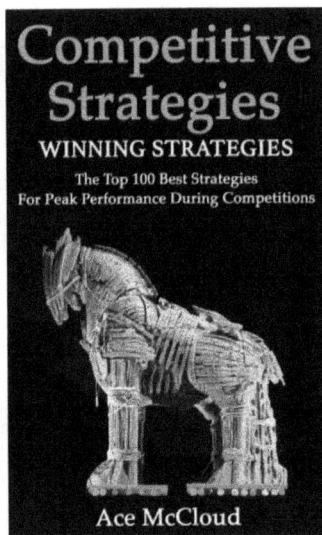

Be sure to check out my audio books as well!

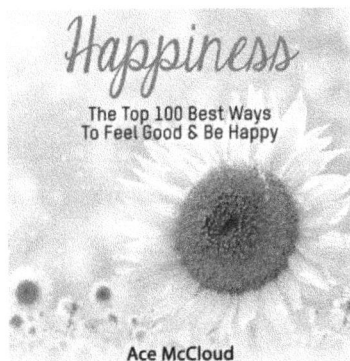

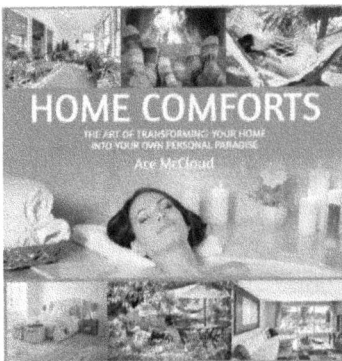

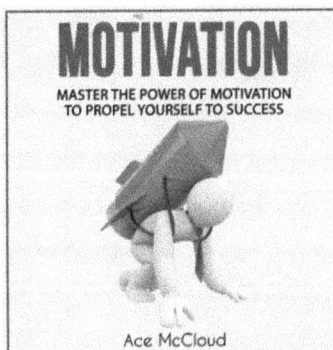

Happiness

The Top 100 Best Ways To Feel Good & Be Happy

Ace McCloud

HOME COMFORTS

THE ART OF TRANSFORMING YOUR HOME INTO YOUR OWN PERSONAL PARADISE

Ace McCloud

MOTIVATION

MASTER THE POWER OF MOTIVATION TO PROPEL YOURSELF TO SUCCESS

Ace McCloud

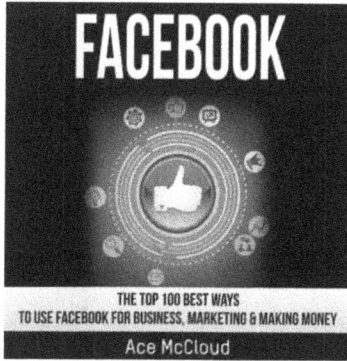

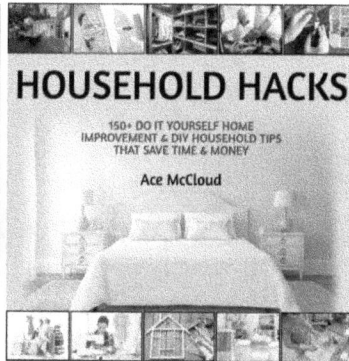

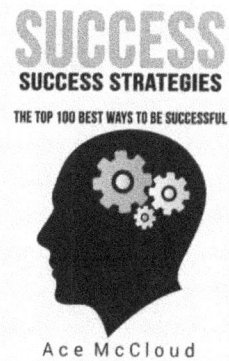

Check out my website at: **www.AcesEbooks.com** for a complete list of all of my books and high quality audio books. I enjoy bringing you the best knowledge in the world and wish you the best in using this information to make your journey through life better and more enjoyable! **Best of luck to you!**

www.ingramcontent.com/pod-product-compliance
Lightning Source LLC
Chambersburg PA
CBHW080632030426
42336CB00018B/3174